Get Up and Move Your A**!

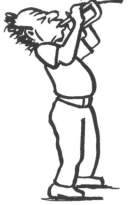

A
Light-Hearted
But Serious
Guide to
Successful Aging

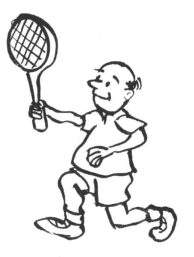

By Patricia Bloom, MD and
Harrison Bloom, MD

illustrations by Isabella Bannerman

Dedication

To Jane, and in memory of Paul, Percy, and Norman, our parents who inspired us by their vigorous lifestyles

and

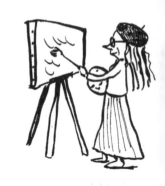

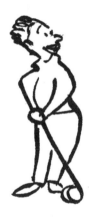

To Laura, Ryan, and Quinn and Jenny, Jedd, and Liliana, our kids and grandkids who give us lots of reasons to stay healthy and active

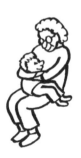

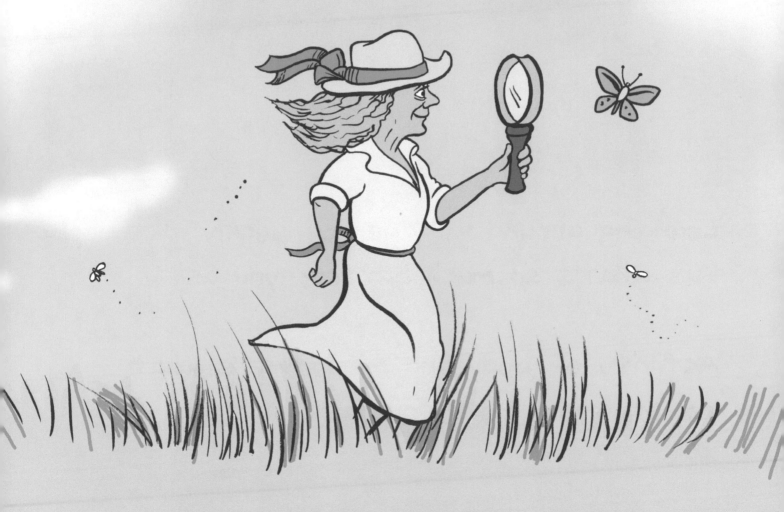

Your 40s, 50s, maybe 60s have passed
So what, you've nothing to dread
There's plenty to do, experience, learn
If you just get your ass out of bed

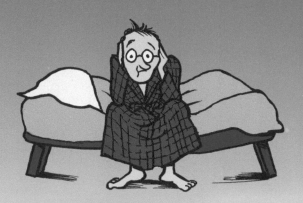

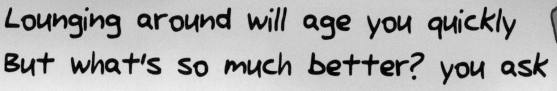

Lounging around will age you quickly
But what's so much better? you ask

Activity of body and mind, that's what
You have to move your ass

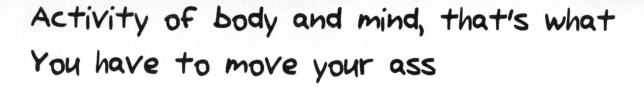

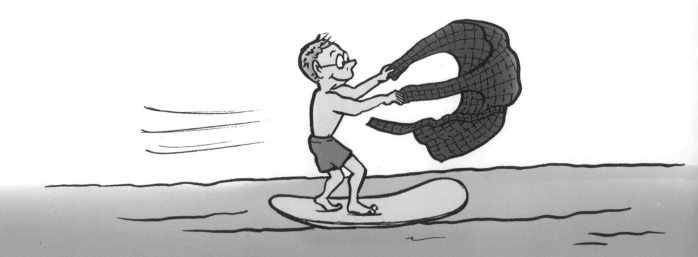

30 minutes of moving around
Research proves benefit,
go ahead

Swim it,
walk it,
bike it,
dance it

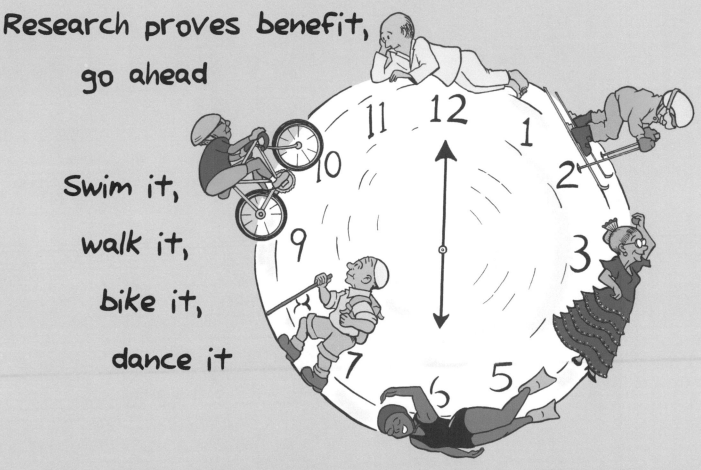

But first get your ass out of bed

A colorful palette upon your plate
Paints a scene of sound body and head

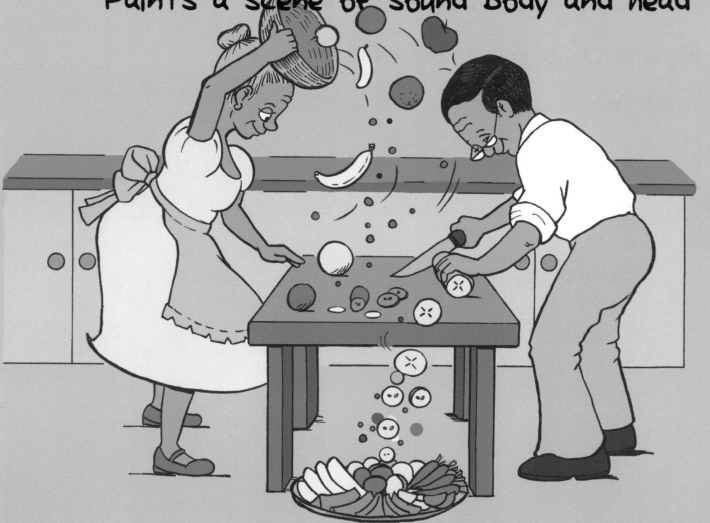

So rise and shine, fruits and veggies in mind
As you get your ass out of bed

4

Wash your face, bathe, and comb your hair
Get dressed, attend a class

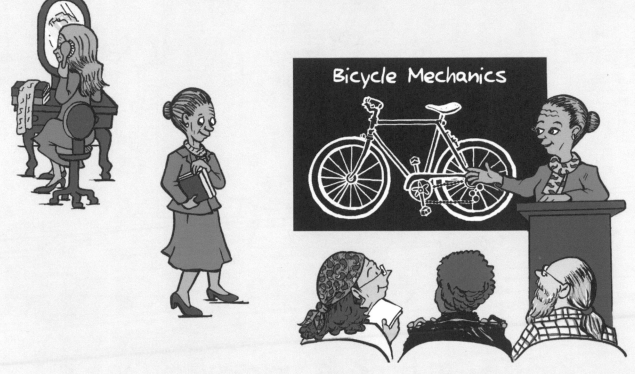

You'll learn a lot, contribute as well,
So out of bed, move your ass!

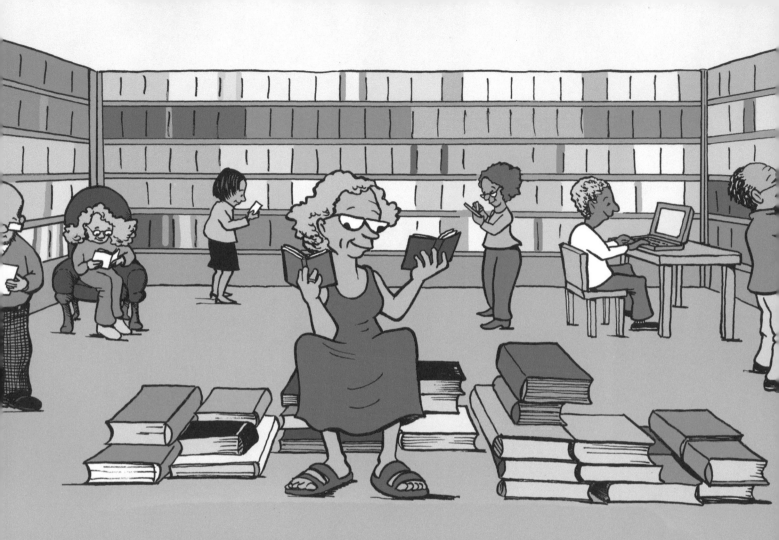

Reading a book, a journal or paper
Perhaps to poetry you're wed
Even going on-line can reward
So get your ass out of bed

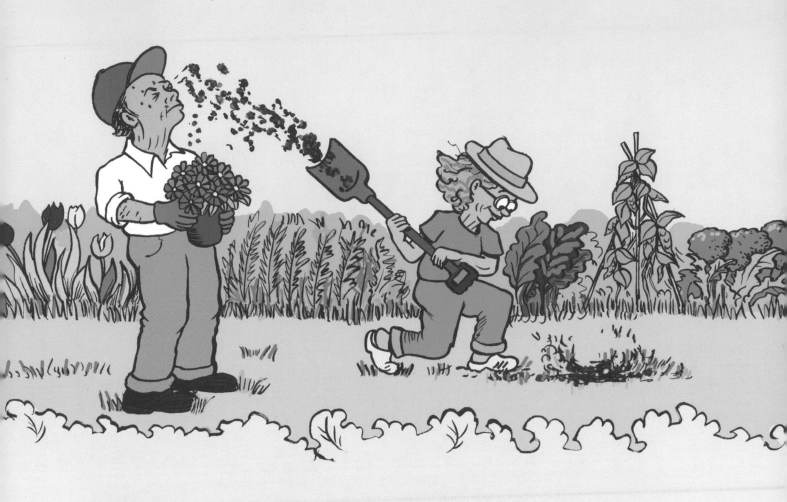

Gardening brings an abundance of life
Tools are ready in the shed
Veggies will grow, flowers will bloom
If you get your ass out of bed

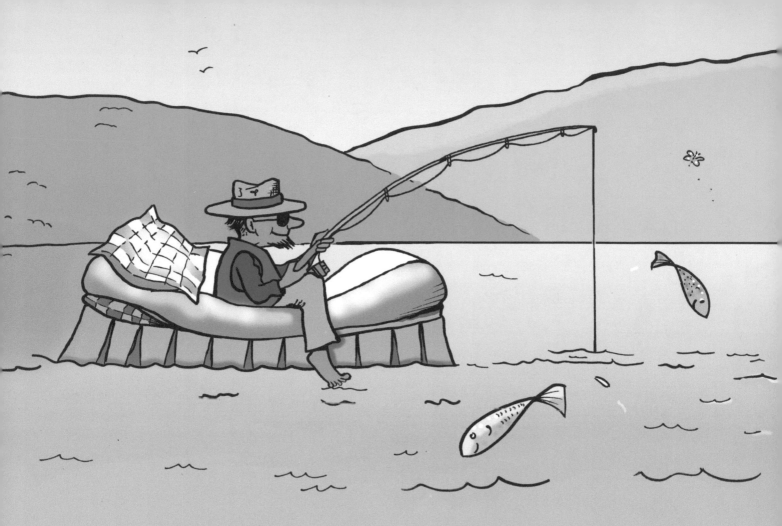

Used to love fishing in rivers and lakes
Catching trout, big walleye and bass?
Can't do that while lying in bed
So get out, move your ass

Use a cane or walker?
If so, quite slowly you tread

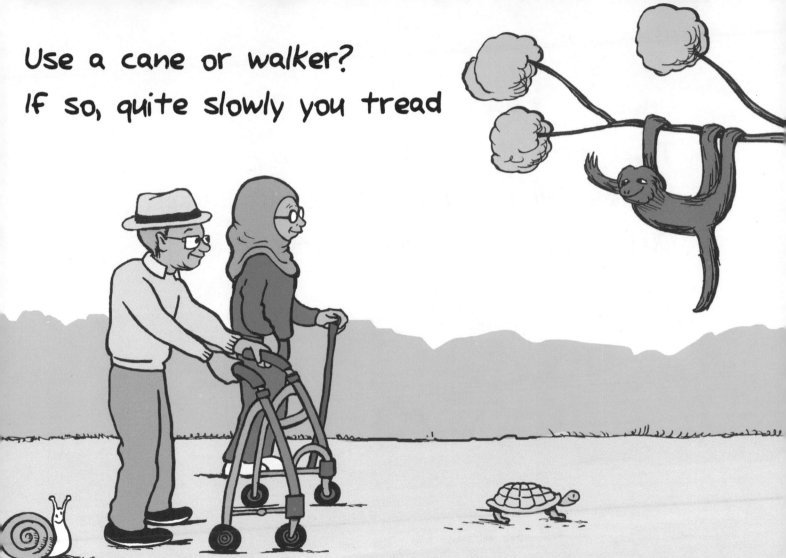

That's fine, no rush, no worries
Just get your ass out of bed

Used to sing or play piano?
That provided lots of fun
Notes will return, just start again
Out of bed now, move your bum

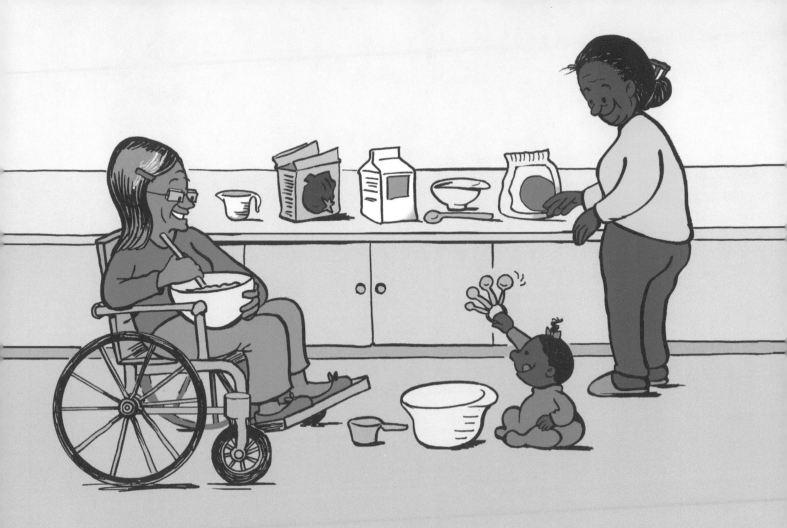

You're quite the cook and baker
So your family have said
Make something fresh and yummy
But first get out of bed

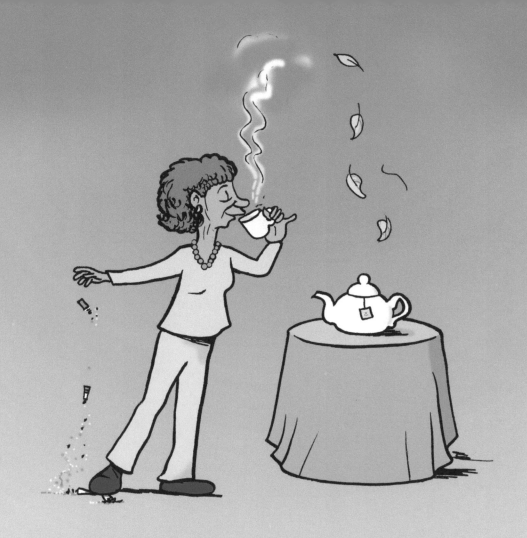

If smoking remains a daily habit
Go drink some green tea instead
Throw those coffin nails into the trash
And you won't burn your ass in bed

Still interested in having sex?
That's great! Now don't feel glum
Intimacy with friend or self
That'll make you move your bum

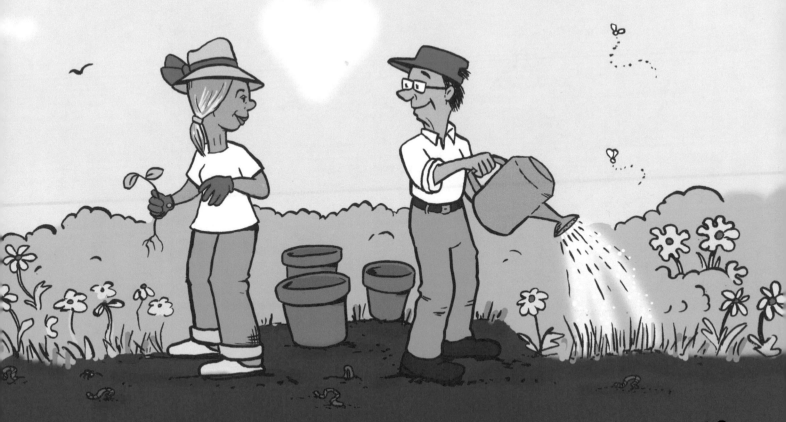

If you enjoy a nice nap, that's fine
45 minutes (or so) it should last

Then open your eyes and dangle your legs
Now get up, move your ass

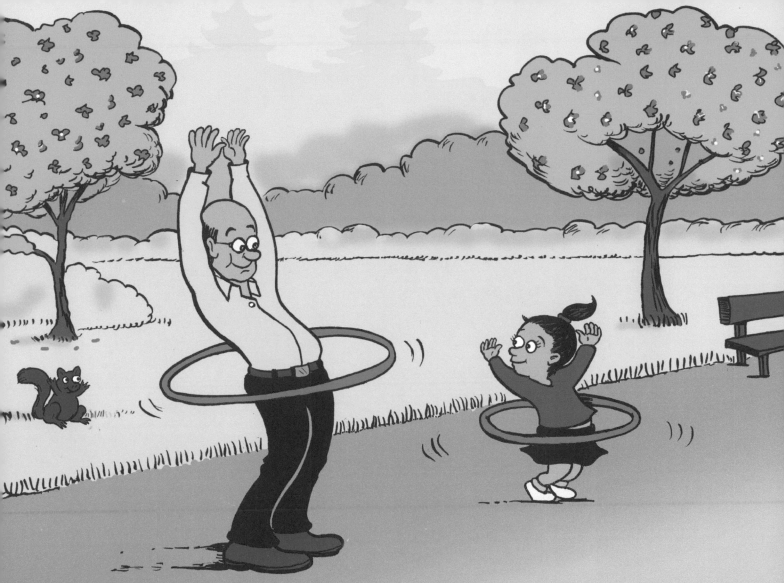

Socializing with kids of all ages is great
Go on and have some fun!
Do something silly, new and wild
Get going, move your bum

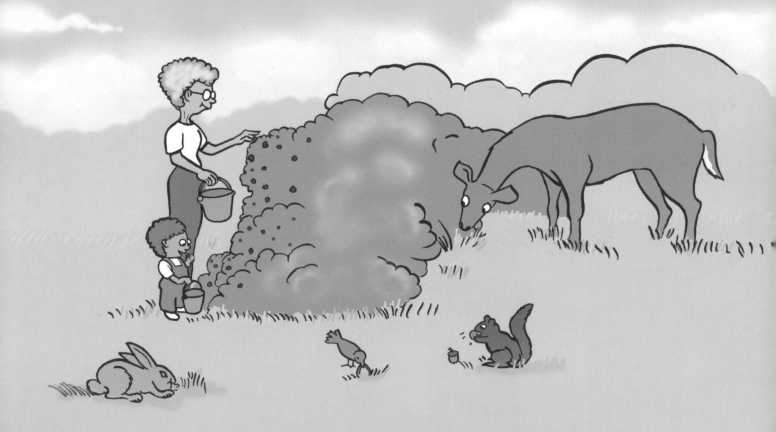

Activity, fiber, hydration
All are a boon to your gut

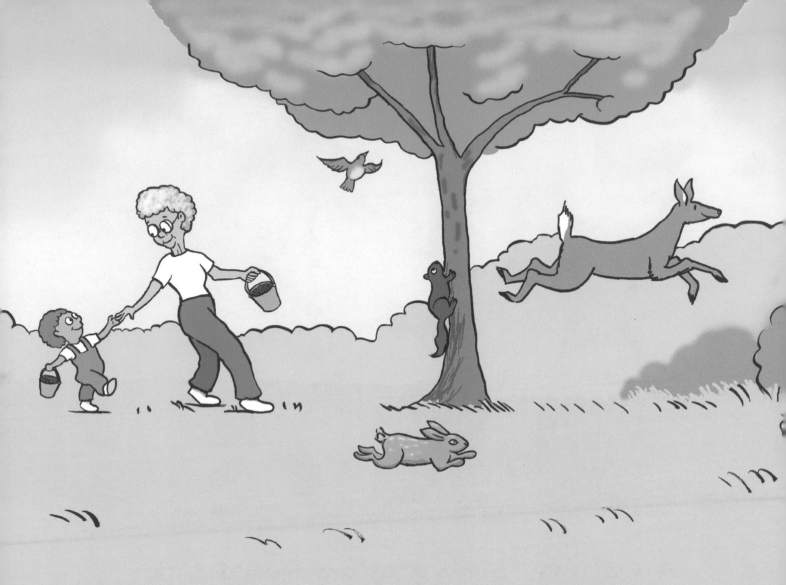

You can keep yourself nicely regular
If you move and get off your butt

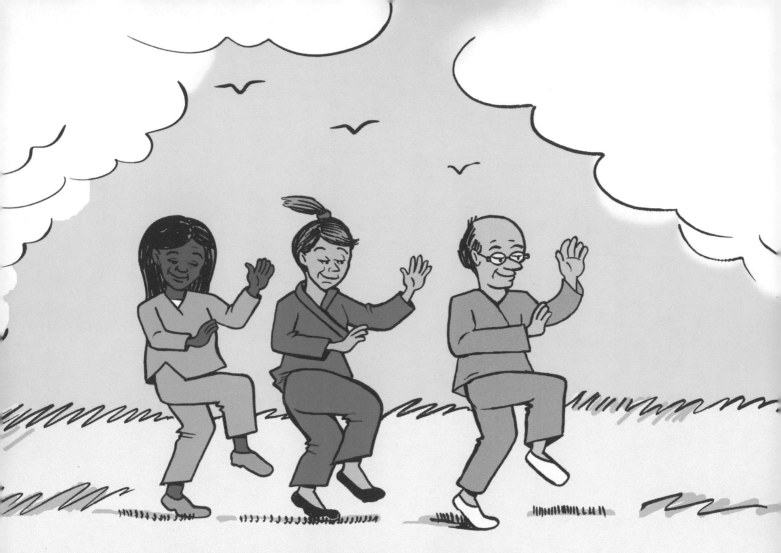

A fall may begin the downward slide
Toward running out of gas
So exercise, balance, do tai chi
And you therefore won't fall on your ass

18

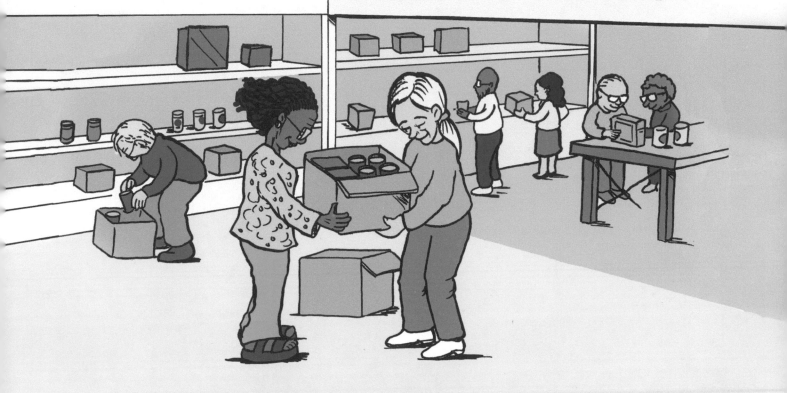

Generosity opens your heart
Feeds body, soul, and head
Random acts of kindness, helping out
Mean you won't get your butt stuck in bed

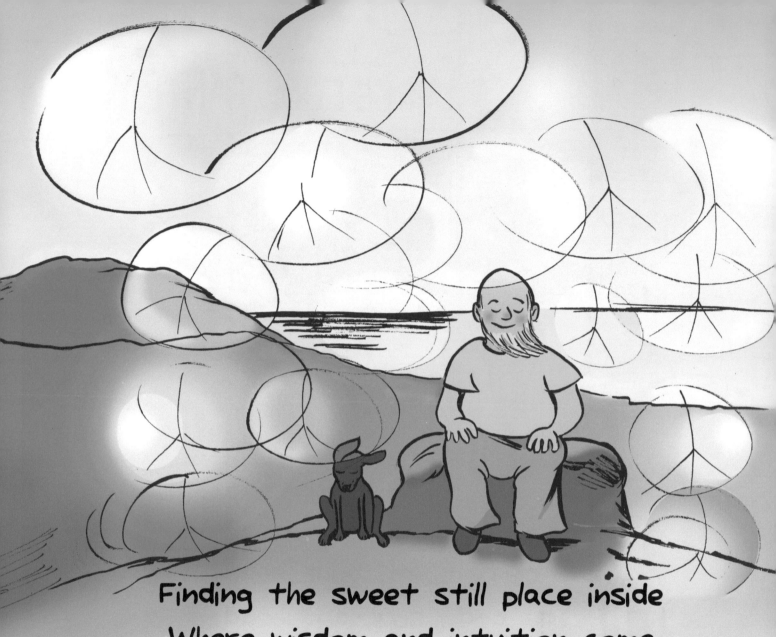

Finding the sweet still place inside
Where wisdom and intuition come
Prayer, meditation, yoga, a walk
Can lead there, you bet your bum

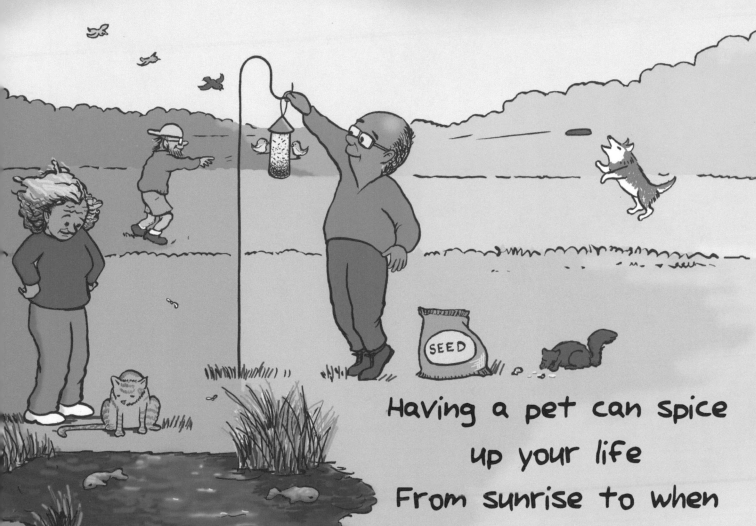

Having a pet can spice
up your life
From sunrise to when
day is done
Great companions for
fun, love and play
They'll insure that you must move your bum

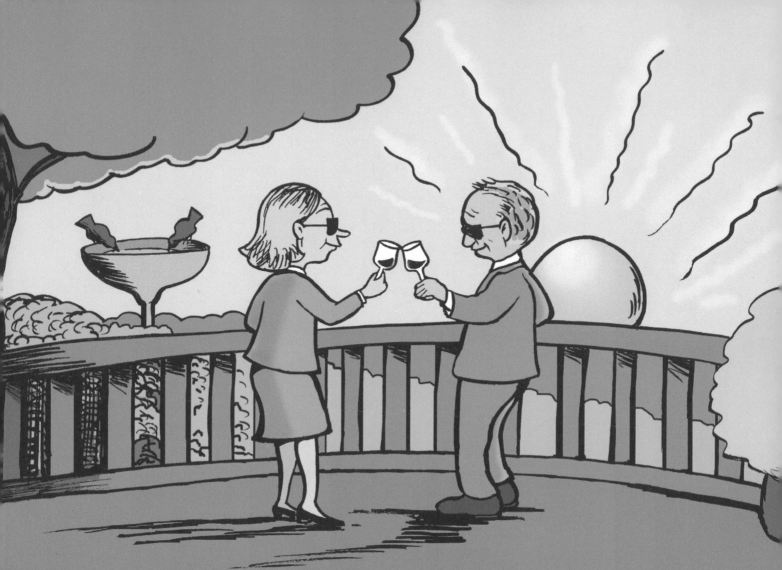

Enjoying a drink as the sun goes down?
No one should say "Tut, tut"
If you limit yourself to one as you sip
It's good for your heart and your butt

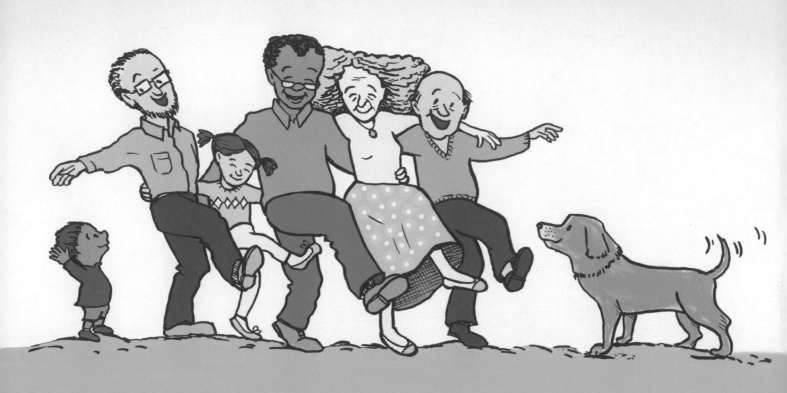

Gratitude for all you have
Is known to benefit your head
Give thanks for family, friends, and stuff
And that you <u>can</u> get your ass out of bed

Ah sleep! 7 or 8 hours the ideal
Time for body and mind to retread
Warm bath, soft tunes, room dark and cool
Sweet dreams, get your ass INTO bed

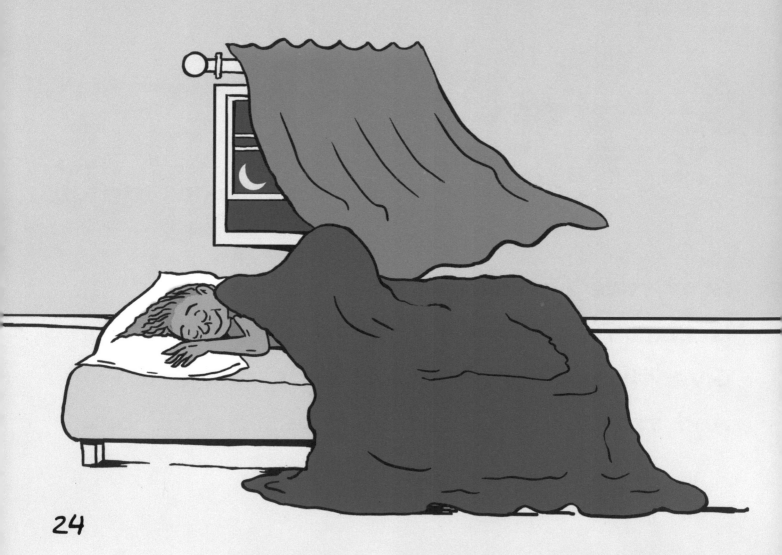

If light-hearted tips leave you skeptical
And wanting some more of the facts
Then check out this science and data
To confirm why you should move your ass

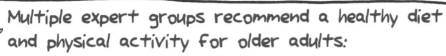

Multiple expert groups recommend a healthy diet and physical activity for older adults:

- American Geriatrics Society: HealthinAging.org
- National Institute on Aging: Exercise & Physical Activity: Your Everyday Guide from the National Institute on Aging. January, 2015

- U.S. Preventive Services Task Force (www.uspreventiveservicestaskforce.org)
- U.S. Department of Health and Human Services. 2008 Physical Activity Guidelines for Americans.

"Exercise is roughly the only equivalent of a fountain of youth that exists today, and it's free to everyone."

-Dr. Jay Olshansky, leading aging expert
"Science (and Quacks) vs. the Aging Process," NYTimes, Nov. 19, 2014

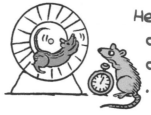

Healthy lifestyle (physical activity 30+min/day, healthy diet, not smoking, moderate alcohol) predicts less heart disease, cancer, diabetes, stroke, and death:

- Akesson, Weismayer, Newby, Wolk. Arch Intern Med 2007;167(19):2122-2127
- Chiuve, McCullough, Sacks. Circulation 2006;114(2):160-7.
- Gorelick. Circulation 2008;118:904-906.
- Hoevenaar-Blom, Spijkerman, Kromhout. Eur J Prev Cardiol 2014. 21(11):1367-75. (includes 7+ hours of sleep per night which further reduced risk of heart attack)
- Hu, Manson, Stampfer. NEJM 2001; 345(11):790-7.
- Knoops, deGroot, Kromhout. JAMA 2004;292:1433-39.

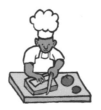

Physical activity, diet, and risk of dementia:

- Barberger-Gateau, Raffaitin, Letenneur. Neurology 2007;69:1921-30.
- Buchman, Boyle, Yu. Neurology 2012; 78:1323-29.
- Etgen, Sander, Huntgeburth. Arch Intern Med 2010;170(2):186-93.
- Larson, Wang, Bowen. Ann Intern Med 2006;144:73-81.
- Scarmeas, Luchsinger, Mayeux. Neurology 2007;69:1084-93.
- Scarmeas, Luchsinger, Schupf. JAMA 2009;302(6):627-37.

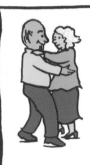

Sexuality in older adults:
- Butler, Lewis. The New Love and Sex After 60. Ballantine Books, NY. 2002.

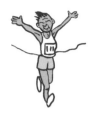

Smoking and longevity:
- Taylor, Hasselblad, Henley. Am J Publ Health 2002;92:990-96.

Social support and wellbeing:
- Berkman, Syme. Am J Epidemiol 1979;109(2):186-204.
- Giles, Glonek, Luszcz. J Epidemiol Community Health 2005;59(7):574-79.
- Holt-Lunstad, Smith, Baker. Perspectives on Psych Sci 2015;10(2):227-37.
- Rasulo, Christensen, Tomassini. Gerontologist 2005;45(5):601-08.